101 Easy Things to do for a Loved One with Cancer

101 Easy Things to do for a
Loved One with Cancer

Cynthia Luane Sleeper

Writers Club Press
San Jose New York Lincoln Shanghai

101 Easy Things to do for a Loved One with Cancer

Writers Club Press
an imprint of iUniverse, Inc.

For information address:
iUniverse, Inc.
5220 S. 16th St., Suite 200
Lincoln, NE 68512
www.iuniverse.com

ISBN: 0-595-21670-6

Printed in the United States of America

Contents

101 Easy Things to do for a Loved One with Cancer

I spent my whole life being the strong one, super woman. Putting everyone's needs ahead of my own and trying to be the best wife, daughter, sister, employee I could be. I organized every event and volunteered time I didn't really have, just like my mother had done. It always seem to come easier for her. She could fit more into a twenty-four hour day than anyone I've ever met. She also had an inner strength and strong faith in God to keep her going when she was tired, hurting, or overwhelmed. She and my father adopted a special needs child when she was 10 months old and she is the sparkle in our families eyes. My father taught me to have a strong work ethic. I love a challenge and had never turned down a project or a new task.

I had a pretty hard year, lost my mother quite suddenly, my brother attempted suicide and will be permanently disabled for the rest of his life. The police came and told my parents my brother had dived from two stories up and landed on his head. They did not expect him to survive the surgery. My older sister came and took my little sister to her house to free up my parents to go to the hospital. My mom wanted to say a prayer over my brother before he went into surgery, but due to a paper work snafu they would not allow this. My mom collapsed and was admitted. They discovered one of her main arteries was about to burst, and were prepping her for surgery but God took her before they were able to operate. I've never worried about her, I know she went on the express train to Heaven and I feel she poured her life's blood into my brother and he pulled through the surgery. I was out of the country teaching when I got pulled off a plane and was given the news that my mother had passed away and my brother would most likely be gone by the time I could arrange to fly home.

The family waited until I was able to fly home; which was quite an adventure of its' own. We then met at the folks house and explained to my little sister about moms' passing. We then made the memorial arrangements, and continued to visit my brother in ICU who was in coma and they were unsure if he was brain dead. I'll never forget our visit to the funeral home trying to plan two services at once. Thank God my brother survived, although he did not come out of the coma for a couple of weeks, so he knew nothing of moms passing.

It was decided that my husband and I would bring my little sister to our house and raise her. I was so overwhelmed with this decision. My husband and I had chosen many years ago not to have children. I travel for my job and never saw the glory of motherhood that so many women speak of. I'm great with pets, and I loved having a little sister, but 24x7 scarred me to death. I'd been the baby of the family for 40 years and my sister is a kindergarten teacher, she got the kids gene. We stopped by the mailbox after picking up a few things my little sister would need and the three of us entered the house for the first time as a family.

I saw in the mail a notice that there was some concern with my recent mammogram and they'd like me to come in for an ultra sound. Some how I knew immediately that I had cancer. I've always been an optimist, but with our family history of cancer and some unknown source within told me it was cancer. In retrospect I feel the timing was perfect because we changed our plans. Dad sold the family home and had a new home built with 6 bedrooms. My cousin, her husband and their son moved in with my father and little sister and have created a wonderful home life for not only my sister but for my dad too. I thank God everyday that my cousin was there for us. She was made to raise children and she has all the skills I am lacking when in comes to motherhood.

In addition to my mothers passing, dealing with cancer, my brothers slow recovery and imminent divorce and trial, along with child raising issues, my mother in law had a aneurism in her stomach burst which caused her to fall into a comma. My husband flew back east to meet with his siblings to decide if they should disconnect her from life support. The day before this was to happen, my husband and his brother spent the entire day by her side in the hospital. My husband, who once worked at a nursing home, explained to his unconscious mother exactly what had occurred over the last two months and the plans they had for her. She suddenly opened her eyes and slowly came out of her coma. She continued to incur many small strokes and we've had to put her in a nursing home.

On top of all that, my soon to be "EX" sister-in-law was calling us all in the middle of the night to say horrible things. Besides all this my father and brother-in-law came to blows over child care decisions. My life start to feel like I was living in a soap opera!

After my tests, they decided I needed a biopsy, which confirmed that I had breast cancer. I went through two surgeries in two weeks and the doctors got it all. This was followed by radiation and I'm now on oral chemotherapy for the next five years. This had caused a few side effects which caused a third surgery, a radical hysterectomy nine months after the other surgeries. I feel I've learned so many life lessons through cancer. It helped me to come to terms with losing one of my closest friends, my mom. I feel if she could have listened to her body once in a while she might still be here with us. I'm still learning that some times you need to put yourself first in order to be the best wife, friend, worker, or person you can be. I've improved my eating and exercising routines, and most importantly I realize how precious life is and who I can really depend on in times of trouble.

I came up with lots of great ideas that helped get me through the steps, like treating radiation as a date by always getting dressed nice and putting on makeup for each visit. I scheduled lunch dates at important mile stones along the way and scheduled a great vacation for a few weeks after my treatments were completed. I found a wonderful devotional for cancer patients with three pages of reading for each day. I'd get to my appointment a little early, put on my lovely white gown and read the devotion. It always seems to say just what I needed to hear on that particular day.

I went to a couple of support groups, read every book I could get my hands on, drove my oncologist nuts with questions, perused the Internet to learn as much as I could about each new process I went through. I'm now involved in a new program where they buddy up a cancer survivor with a newly diagnosed person. I've found this to be so rewarding by learning that we all have different fears, concerns, questions, needs and that different doctors have very different approaches to attacking this disease. No two peoples' paths through cancer are the same.

I lost contact with so many friends, family members and co-workers who were either frightened by the word CANCER, or were just clueless as to how they could help.

This book will hopefully give people ideas that will work so you can feel like you're a part of your friends or loved ones healing process. I learned that it was important for my friends to help, that it wasn't imposing on them. They actually felt better once I *quit* saying "Oh no, I'm fine, I've got everything covered."

Dedication

I dedicate this book to God and his infinite wisdom, my wonderful supportive husband, Mark without whom I'd never have seen the light at the end of the tunnel. My husband and I have been together over 25 years and have made it through some tough times before, but I fell in love all over again with the man he became when I needed him most.

I've been blessed through out my life to have a best friend since I was three and a half years old. Marybeth, was there everyday doing things for me, calling to check on me, stopping at the store, pharmacy or video store to pick up items I needed and most importantly encouraging me. I'm forever in her debt.

Idea Number One

Get a list of favorite movies that are out on video that your friend would like to see. Pick up one a week and drop it by, maybe even stay and watch it with them. Take it upon yourself to pickup the tape and return it. Verify if they own a VCR or a DVD.

The local library has several classics that can be checked out for no cost. These videos can be checked out for several weeks. This will allow your friend to watch the movie at their leisure.

Several video stores sell their extra copies of a movie after it has been released for a couple of months. These films are sold at a much lower price that new video copies. Purchasing a copy can be a great option when there are children in the household.

Idea Number Two

Several video stores have a card that gives a discount for multiple rentals. For example 30 videos in 30 days. This forces the person to take some down time. It is amazing how many cancer survivors are workaholic. I found it very hard to rest each afternoon even for an hour. During chemotherapy and radiation the body seems to tire out a bit more each day. So many things don't get done. The down side to this is when you're feeling good you over do trying to catch up. I made this mistake many times. It takes a couple of days to recover when you push past that imaginary line. It is imperative while going through these exhausting procedures to take this downtime every day and reevaluate the "To do list".

Idea Number Three

Send a postcard or a small note in the mail once a week or so. This is really great if the patient needs a lot of rest. You can be assured you're not waking them up, but they know you're thinking of them. I looked so forward to the mail each day. I had a co-worker who made a point of mailing me a little note every couple of days while I was on disability. My husband put all the cards I received up on my closet doors. By the time I returned to work, my bedroom was wall to wall cards. Cancer makes you feel alone sometimes; these constant reminders that someone is thinking of you can be really uplifting.

Idea Number Four

People who have children and are going through surgeries, chemotherapy and/or radiation need even more help. Offer to take the kids to and from an event or to school. Plan a special day with the kids where you go to a movie, or park, walk on the beach. Help them with their homework. Most kids have after school sports or other activities that they need rides to and from. Take them shopping. We all have a special skill; take time to teach a child how to play an instrument, do an arts and craft project, make a card or cook dinner together for mom.

Take the kids out with a disposable camera and let them take pictures of favorite places or of each other playing at the park, in a softball game, swimming, whatever. Then have the film developed and share the day with their mom or dad that's stuck at home.

Idea Number Five

Offer to watch the kids or feed them once a week. Find out what time radiation is each day and stay with the kids during this time. Better yet find out what time they get home after their daily radiation and be there to watch the kids and answer the phone while they lie down for an hour.

Idea Number Six

Drop off dinner, or their favorite snack. This was a big treat for me. I would have never asked anyone to bring me dinner, but when they did it anyway, I was so touched. This took a big load off my husband too. He'd work all day then come home and try and do things around the house before I could get to them. He says I'm the worlds worst patient. He learned how to do several things around the house that he'd never done. We've been together over 20 years. I had no idea he was so capable around the house. When someone would bring a meal it meant he could get to other things or spend more time with me.

Idea Number Seven

Make a lunch date with your friend once a week during chemotherapy or radiation. Make sure they know it's ok to back out at the last minute. Keep in mind some people can't eat spicy foods or large quantities during treatments. Just driving them to treatment and bringing a picnic lunch is fun too. Go to a park or the beach and sit and eat while you talk or enjoy the scenery.

Idea Number Eight

E-mail jokes or e-cards to their account. The great thing about e-mail is the recipient can read it when they feel like it. It's not like a phone call that might wake them up. There are several web sites that have e-cards that you just have to add your name to and send. Doesn't take long and they're great fun to receive. The variety is amazing, there are some with sound bytes, some animated, some interactive.

Idea Number Nine

Ask what would be the best time to call and set up a specific day of the week or time that works for them. So many people are afraid to call so they lose touch. Quite often when going through cancer treatments people are homebound more than they're accustom to. This causes a feeling of isolation. Setting up a time to expect a call makes it easier for you to follow through and gives your friend something to look forward to. I wanted to be in the know about what was going on in the office. I had a couple of co-workers who would call me on Fridays to clue me in on what I was missing. If you are a manager with someone on disability going through cancer treatments set up a weekly or bi-weekly call. Let them know their job is there waiting for them, encourage them, don't rush them back.

Idea Number Ten

Go with them to a support group the first time so they feel empowered. Use the yellow pages or check with their Oncologist or local Hospice for a list of groups. I was amazed how many different types of cancer support groups are out there. There are groups that meet at churches that sing and pray and share what they're going through. There are groups that specialize on learning everything they can about cancer and the different treatments.

There are alternative groups that use your mind, with yoga, acupuncture, art or other philosophies to deal with cancer. There are sexual preference and sexual difficulty support groups. The most important part is meeting with people that have or are going through the same things your loved one is dealing with.

I belonged to a support group through the church at first and I'm now in a new program called Navigator. We are funded partially by the tobacco tax and Stanford University is compiling information we gather to determine if having support improves the lives of cancer survivors. The oncologist in our area explains the program to newly diagnosed patients. If the patient chooses, they can become a sojourner and will be matched to a navigator who has experienced a similar type of cancer. Both sojourner and navigator fill out paperwork describing what attributes are most important in a match. We have a specialist who does a great job of matching. I've worked with five sojourners and have learned so much, made some new friends and hopefully helped them through a difficult time.

Sometimes cancer patients don't want to burden their loved ones with all the things they're going through. There were times when cancer was all I thought about and could have talked about it non-stop. I liked being able to talk to people who weren't in my day to day life and wouldn't feel my pain, fear, anger, or sorrow like my loved ones would have if I shared with them. I'm not saying you shouldn't talk to your friend about what they're going through, but understand some things they can't share with you and some things you just can't help with until you've walked in their shoes.

Idea Number Eleven

Take on a chore, don't take no for an answer. Vacuum the house once a week, polish the furniture, water the house plants, sweep and mop the kitchen or catch up with the laundry. Find out what is getting under their skin around the house or yard. I can't stand dirty dishes or trash in my waste paper baskets. My best friend knew this and would take care of these things when ever she came by. Make sure you respect your friend. Some people take it as a sign of weakness when they can't do everything for themselves. Work with them to clean up a room, force them to take breaks. Make it fun. Teach their kids or husband how they can help.

Idea Number Twelve

Pick up their prescriptions or vitamins for them. It seemed like I was constantly running out of something. I went from taking nothing to taking a handful of pills twice a day. There are several vitamins necessary to counteract the treatments. Make sure they are aware of these requirements. In working with several cancer patients I've found that each oncologist shares different information with their patients.

Sometimes if you don't ask, the doctors don't even get into things like taking an aspirin every day while on oral chemotherapy, or the need for higher doses of vitamin C and E while going through radiation. There are so many great books that explain the reasons for each vitamin and the necessary doses to take during and after treatments.

Idea Number Thirteen

Change the bed sheets. Seems like I spent half my day in bed for a while there, especially after the surgeries. Nothing feels better than clean sheets. What's really fun is to run a bath with special smelling bubbles. Check with them first, they might not be able to take a bath right after surgery or during radiation. You change the sheets while they're in the bath. Shake a little baby powder on the mattress before you put the bottom sheet on. Really makes them smell nice. Scent the light bulbs using aroma therapy scents that create calm or healing. Add some fresh flowers to the room. Buy a new comforter that they can drag from the bed to the recliner to the chaise lounge outside.

Idea Number Fourteen

Supply small fun gifts, flowers or candles. Make sure smells don't effect them first. Gifts from the office or their kids are especially nice. It is important to know who is aware of their cancer. Some people choose to keep this a secret so they don't have to go back to work and answer questions or get treated differently. Some people even worry about losing their jobs or possible promotions. The decision on whom to tell is solely up the patient. Make sure you honor this.

There is a product called Fuzzy Art, it is a poster that comes with five colored markers. I found these to be so much fun. It's something they can do with their kids or by themselves. It forces a person to take some down time, create and relax. Crossword puzzles, favorite magazines, local newspapers, embroidery, craft kits, coloring book and crayons. The list is endless, be creative. Find out what they enjoy and bring them some silly little thing each time you come by. I love presents, so therefore anything I get to unwrap cheers me up.

Idea Number Fifteen

Drop off books from the library or books you've bought that are uplifting, informative, or just distracting. There are some really great books out there about dealing with Cancer. I've changed so much since my experience. You change your priorities in life. Books are my drug of choice. I read everything I could get my hands on when I first got diagnosed. Some people like to read about the different options before they have to make the big decisions. I found the books useful when side effects popped up. Most of these books have recommendations to bring up with your Oncologist.

Some people don't like to read or they can't handle reading about cancer. Talk to your friend about what kind of books they like, bring up a list from the Times or the Internet and let them circle the ones they'd like to read. Read the book at the same time so you can discuss it with them. Take them to the library or book store with you so they can pick out a book for themselves.

Idea Number Sixteen

Offer to take them to their appointments or go with them. Sometimes the doctor gives so much information that you leave the appointment wishing you'd taped it. So go ahead take a cassette player and tape the appointments. Make a list of all the drugs they take and the dose. If the doctor prescribes anything new remind them what your friend is already taking. This can reduce the side effects. Doctors see a lot of people everyday and I've learned they don't remember as much about me as I'd always thought. It's important for a cancer survivor to become their own advocate. You can make up a big folder or file and help them organize copies of doctors notes, x-rays, test results and keep a calendar of who they saw when. Having a copy of their records reduces wasted appointments. Quite often the doctor doesn't have your x-ray or the latest mammogram results or recent blood test. I found this frustrating. In creating your own cancer files your able to keep this from happening and can answer unexpected questions that come up regarding previous test, surgeries or drug allergies.

Idea Number Seventeen

Insist on driving once a week to radiation. Great chance to visit and doesn't interfere with when they might be resting. It was unbelievable to me how big of a chunk of time this seemed to take. Forty treatments, five days a week same time every day. Nice to shake it up so take a different route each time you drive them. Borrow a friends convertible. I saw so many people dragging themselves in and out of treatment. I really think your mind set makes a huge difference.

Idea Number Eighteen

Go for walks, pick new and unusual places. Make sure you are near a phone or have your cellular phone with you. Bring water and plan short walks. Half hour walks are great. I loved taking my dog with us and giving her a little outing also. I live in California and was shocked by how many cool places there are to see. Flower gardens, waterfalls, beaches with beautiful cliffs with trees overhanging. It's fun to go where there are a lot of people to watch too.

Idea Number Nineteen

During the holiday season or birthdays offer to pick up the gifts they wanted to purchase, or drive them, or wrap them, or deliver them. Help them with their Christmas cards. I had my third surgery in November and I was overwhelmed with the holidays coming up. Make it easy for them. Get Christmas list for each child so all they have to do is pick up the item. Call around and get prices and availability of the item. Set up their computer with bookmarks where they can shop on line to find the toys, books, or other gifts. This way they can personalize their shopping without ever leaving their house.

Discuss with the family alternatives to reduce big productions, even if it's something you do every year. Use this year to try something different. Keep it simple. Buy a tree and decorate it, then surprise them with it. Remember you need to think of these things before they have a chance to do it themselves.

Idea Number Twenty

Help the other family members too. Give them a night off, or be a shoulder to lean on. Sometimes I think cancer is harder on the family than the person going through it. Sometimes I could see my husband was so tired when he got home from work, yet he'd try to take care of things for me. Pretty soon he'd get a cold or his back would go out. It's important that they have time for themselves too. Do things to try and make life normal for the entire family.

Idea Number Twenty-One

Offer to drive them to their church or other committees they belong to. It is so easy to become incognito when your on disability. I wasn't suppose to drive for a month and half. The only time I got to go somewhere was when I had a ride. Anything is more fun when someone goes with you.

Idea Number Twenty-Two

Come by and water or weed in the yard; they might be able to sit outside and visit with you while you're working. Take their children to a plant store and pick up some soil and a few pretty flowers, or bulbs or a tree. Plant them as a tribute plant them as a tribute. Then they'll be able to enjoy them when they grow and bloom. This can be especially poignant if the patient is terminal. Make a funky sign for the garden or a special rock with an inscription.

Idea Number Twenty-Three

Help with the trash on trash night. It is amazing how many people have to drag a can or two up a hill or down a long driveway. Even when there are other family members it just doesn't get done. You can also retrieve and put the cans back where they belong when you come by and see them still out at the end of the drive. Help with recycling, this can take some time to sort and purge.

Idea Number Twenty-Four

Help them use a camcorder to record messages to their loved ones. Video journals are also fun. It is cool to look back and see how far you've come. Make a funny short film of the patients hobby or favorite subject. Keep it light and fun.

Idea Number Twenty-Five

Clean the bathrooms. The things that are crazy are the things that aren't done, but they can't seem to get through doing themselves. Think about what you would want done if you were stuck in the house and had to stare at four walls day after day. These things are different for everyone, but concentrate on the rooms they tend to spend the most time in.

Idea Number Twenty-Six

Learn something new with them. This can be an online class, a craft, an adult night class or weekend class. Calligraphy, painting, make a photo calendar together. Take a photography class, stain glass, jewelry making. The possibilities are endless. Learn a foreign language then when the treatments are completed, visit that country.

Idea Number Twenty-Seven

Take a yoga class together. I found I couldn't exercise during certain stages of my recovery. My best friend brought me a wonderful beginning yoga tape. I would do this every morning. It really helped. It keeps you limber, helps your mental attitude, and keeps you active.

Idea Number Twenty-Eight

Have them keep a running list of groceries or supplies they need and stop by once a week with the supplies. This includes putting them away once you bring them in. Help their mates plan menus, then create a grocery list based on these meals. Remember lots of fruits and vegetables, proteins and their favorite things.

Idea Number Twenty-Nine

Help with paperwork, and returning phone calls. Insurance companies always seem to need copies or additional forms completed. A spreadsheet tracking medical expenses is also useful. Quite often there is more than one insurance company involved and it gets confusing. Tracking your disability pay is helpful too. Keep track of the hours you have submitted to the State. I found once I returned to work part time the State had difficulties determining my disability income.

Idea Number Thirty

When they have a surgery or other procedure that requires time in the hospital don't go visit them in the hospital the first 24 hours. Call their mates or the hospital, after that to find out if they're ready for visitors. If you can get your hands on a maternity hospital gown or bra, these make great gifts for people who've had breast cancer surgery or are going through radiation treatments. Bring a gift, something small. A photo of their kids or pets to look at while they're in the hospital. It is boring in the hospital so bring a TV guide, book, magazines, crossword puzzles, coloring book and crayons, something colorful to look at.

Idea Number Thirty-One

Keep visits short, look for signs of tiring. Make sure to use touch as a way of communicating. So many people shy away from physical contact, as if cancer was contagious. I'd much rather see someone twice a week for 20 minutes than once for an hour. Remember they're trying to look like they feel ok. Look for eyes staying closed a little longer, slumped shoulders, yawning, loss of attention, or if they suddenly aren't doing any of the talking. Sometimes I was so glad someone stopped by I had them stay too long and then I was sore or tired.

Idea Number Thirty-Two

Video tape things you know they would have loved to attend but couldn't. Kids play, trip to the beach, vacation pictures. Have the kids say something special at the beginning of the tape about how much they missed having mom or dad there, or how much they love them. Keep the tape and add to it every time you take the kids for an afternoon or doing something your friend would have enjoyed. Go to the office and video the office. It's comforting to see how little changes while your gone.

Idea Number Thirty-Three

Let them know they can have a pity party sometimes, that everyone gets overwhelmed on occasion. Don't say it will get better, or think of those worst off. Just listen and let them vent. If they seem to stay in a state of depression suggest they tell their oncologist. Quite often anti-depression drugs are required to get through certain rough patches. Depression can also hit after the storm is over. Signs of depression are they're always in bed, don't bother getting dressed or brushing their teeth. Constantly come up with reasons why they can't go out with you. Weight gain or loss can also be signs, but since different cancer treatment drugs cause both weight gain and loss, this is a hard one to diagnose.

Idea Number Thirty-Four

If they continue to work, even part time call them at the office and make sure they take it easy. With cancer treatments you have good days and bad days, slow them down on the good days and encourage them on the bad days. My girlfriend still calls me twice a week to make sure I'm taking my breaks. Sometimes she even comes by the office and we take a walk to the beach.

Idea Number Thirty-Five

If they have a strong faith in God, include them in a prayer chain, and pray with them. There are several great devotionals and books written by Christians with cancer. There is even a news letter and web sites. I found several of these when I need to be uplifted. If they don't have God in their lives maybe now would be a good time to tell them about the Lord. I really don't believe I would have gotten through the last two years without God. I relied on him on a daily sometimes hourly basis.

Idea Number Thirty-Six

There are so many difficult decisions to make in the first couple of weeks after a cancer diagnosis. Help them to research, and seek options. It is not that big of a rush, it is much more important when they look back on these decisions, they're happy with the choices they made. There are literally thousands of resources out there. Utilize them. Check out the library, Internet, support groups. I read several great books that walked me through what to expect during each stage. Don't overwhelm them. Just learn what you need as you need it.

Idea Number Thirty-Seven

Utilize the many resources that are available in your county. I was shocked to find out how many different organizations were out there to help with decisions, money problems, getting to an appointment, or other issues. Use the yellow pages, call the American Cancer Society, their church, or their doctor to obtain a list of support groups and agencies in your area to assist with decisions, emotional support and even financial aid.

Idea Number Thirty-Eight

If you live in the house or work with the person, leave little encouraging notes around to be found unexpectedly. My husband is great about doing this. Every morning when I'd go in to get my morning cup of coffee he'd have drawn a little picture on a piece of paper and left the coffee stirrer on it. I'd go out to my car to drive to radiation and there would be a note on my dashboard. Cancer sometimes made me feel like I wasn't a woman anymore, sometimes I didn't even feel human. These notes could undo all the horrible things that I could think up about myself. Notes promising a date are great fun too. Some examples could be; "I'll bring home a pizza and a movie tonight". "You're in charge of the popcorn."
It doesn't matter what you say, it's just knowing that you're thinking of the person that makes it special. Mark brought me cards, flowers and a new balloon shaped like an animal each week. My bedroom started looking like a zoo. I loved it. He even put up Christmas lights in my bedroom to make it look more lively.

Idea Number Thirty-Nine

Plan a trip, even a day trip or shopping trip. It's nice to have things to look forward to. I scheduled a trip to an all inclusive resort in Cozemel once I knew the date my radiation would end. We had a great time, hung out at the pool, or the pool bar, snorkelled, went on a submarine adventure, had a massage. It was great for both of us. We were ready for a week of rest. I also planned dinners out at my favorite restaurants at key times during radiation and other monumental dates that came up. My friends made dates with me to go out to lunch, go to a play, go shopping for an hour, a day at the spa, walk on the beach, all kinds of wonderful things to look forward to and get my mind off of how I was feeling.

Idea Number Forty

If they can't work, find things they can do to help others when they're up to it. Giving back really uplifts the spirit. Lick envelopes at home for a mailing for a favorite charity or political event. Deliver meals on wheels, read to the children at the library, help out at school one hour a week. I did not feel healed until I was able to go full circle and start giving back. Mentor someone who is going through cancer now and you'll be able to give insight and learn about yourself at the same time.

Idea Number Forty-One

Buy them a journal or make a personalized scrapbook. When I was in pain or couldn't sleep I'd go into my home office and work on my journal. I think better when typing directly into the computer, but many people prefer to write down their thoughts on paper. I've looked back on these writings many times and plan to write a book someday about the day to day dealings of living with cancer. I also wrote down my dreams and best of all I wrote down five blessings in my life everyday.
The more energy I spent thinking of my blessings the less energy I wasted feeling sorry for myself.

Idea Number Forty-Two

Change traditions so they can still participate in some manner but not be overwhelmed. Little things, like instead of buying gifts at Christmas each person will do something for each person. Or instead of getting together for a huge turkey dinner, maybe order Chinese food, or just get together for dessert. I'm lucky enough to work for the best company in the world. They went out of their way to eliminate any responsibilities I would normally have and let us use their beautiful lodge on a lake in Northern California. We spent a very special New Years Eve. This was such a wonderful experience. It allowed us time as a family to talk about what we were all going through and take long walks in the woods, sit by the fire and just relax. This was not the usual hustle and bustle of the holidays.

Idea Number Forty-Three

It seems like cancer is more likely to happen to those who are doers, the ones who are used to fixing things, and helping others. Remember it is a new experience for these types of people to have to ask for help. Chances are they won't. You need to step in and tell them what you're going to do. I discovered that the people who care for me needed to feel useful. Once I opened up and allowed them to help they were able to let go of some of their fears of losing me and they needed to feel like there was something they could do to help.

Idea Number Forty-Four

Make sure they don't feel like they need to hold you up. This was hard for me to learn. I found as soon as my loved one was upset I put my emotions on hold so I could be strong for them. I learned the world doesn't fall apart if your both weak at the same time. In fact it is downright healing to cry about the struggles you're dealing with together.

Idea Number Forty-Five

Tease them, sometimes it all becomes too serious and they just need to laugh. Keep it light, jokes, cartoons anything that makes them laugh. There are studies that show how laughing can really assist in healing the body. I never felt better than when I was laughing, even during the worst of times it makes you forget any aches, pains or hard decision coming up.

Idea Number Forty-Six

If you are a co-worker update them via e-mail or a card on the office gossip or personnel changes. Once a month have them meet you for lunch. It was kind of intimidating returning to work. In retrospect I would have been better off seeing my co-workers a few times while I was on disability. That first day in was pretty scary. Make sure to include them when special events are coming up at the office. Retirements, showers, or anything else.

Idea Number Forty-Seven

Reward them. Make up silly certificates and frame them. These can be for all sorts of milestones such as completion of chemotherapy or radiation. Treat them to a favorite snack, CD of their favorite artist. Anything that tells them you care.

Idea Number Forty-Eight

If they're losing their hair try shaving your head too! There are some really fun temporary tattoos that can be applied. Losing their hair can be one of the hardest things to handle for a cancer patient. Try to prepare them for this possibility and let them know it doesn't effect how beautiful they are. It is a badge of honor, remind them of this as often as required. Take them to a stylist before the hair starts to fall out and come up with a easy to maintain short hair cut. This will reduce the shock of change, if they should experience hair loss.

Idea Number Forty-Nine

Help them pick out a wig. I suggest purchasing the wig before you need it. Remember though that the fit is significantly different when there is no hair to pin up underneath. It is kind of fun to go with a color you've never experienced. They can be a blond or a redhead, have straight or curly hair that they've never experienced.

Idea Number Fifty

Cut your hair and donate it to the "Locks of Love" organization. This wonderful group uses the hair to make wigs for children with cancer. Many salons have connection with these agencies and can handle the arrangements and explain any special requirements. I've seen some of the children who have received these wigs and it is such a wonderful sight.

Idea Number Fifty-One

Get involved in a walk for life or other Cancer funding cause. They have bowling, tennis, softball, and all kinds of events. A cure is right around the corner for this horrible disease. Funding allows for scientific research and also for new drugs to improve the quality of life, help with side effects, and reduce reoccurrence.

Idea Number Fifty-Two

Buy a candle in their name for a cancer fund-raising event. In the evening they light the candles and each one is labeled with the persons name. If they can't go to the event, take a picture and frame it for them. I was so touched at the walk for life when I saw the hundreds of candles lit up. We forget how many lives are touched in every town across the world by cancer. Everyone has a loved one, friend, or co-worker that experiences cancer sometime during their lives.

Idea Number Fifty-Three

Learn more about the type of cancer they have so you have some understanding of what to expect. No two people experience cancer quite the same way. Biopsies, surgery, radiation, and medications effect each of us differently. One procedure might be a walk in the park for them and another will have every complication in the universe. It is amazing how many different side effects the cures for cancer have. Not only physical side effects, but mood swings, memory, sex drive and energy levels are just a few of the areas that can be affected by the treatments and drugs that are given to cancer patients. Make sure they speak up to their doctors about side effects. We sometimes are so grateful to be in remission that we think little problems are a small price to pay. Although this is true, most side effects have cures. Sometimes it is the combination of medications and by changing one drug the side effects will disapear.

Idea Number Fifty-Four

If they don't own a PDR a.k.a. Physicians' Desk Reference book, get them one. There are so many different medications and the doctors don't always keep track of how they interact with another or explain possible side effects. Or which medications you can't take at the same time. Some medications do not interact well with certain vitamins and must be taken at different times during the day.

Idea Number Fifty-Five

Give them a massage, or a coupon for one, or go with them and get one at the same time. Make sure you let the therapist know in advance of any special needs. There are many different types of massages, shop around and find one that best fits your friends needs.

Idea Number Fifty-Six

Look into alternate Eastern ideas like acupuncture, herbal remedies. Try to keep an open mind and a positive outlook. I was sent for sacral cranial therapy and was amazed how much this helped with my residual pain in my chest. There are hundreds of alternatives out there, keep trying until you find the perfect match. Aroma therapy has helped many people with pain and other side effects.

Idea Number Fifty-Seven

Help them to make a list of questions to ask the doctor so they'll remember when they go to their appointments. I purchased a special date book to keep track of appointments, Doctors names and numbers, and any questions and the answers. I still pull this out when it's time to visit my oncologist or surgeon. Every time I go to a Doctors appointment, I'm asked to list the dates of each procedure and where they took place. This special date book has come in handy many times.

Idea Number Fifty-Eight

Purchase cassette tapes for the car. Self help, mind altering or feel good tapes are all great ideas. Cancer patients spend a good deal of time driving back and forth to appointments and procedures. I really enjoyed listening to Bernie S. Siegel, M.D. when I drove to radiation each day. These tapes can also be used while receiving chemotherapy.

Idea Number Fifty-Nine

Alternative head covers are kind of fun. If they are losing their hair look at some beautiful scarfs, or funky hats. I got to the point where I looked forward to seeing what one of my friends would be wearing each time I saw her. Several agencies make a type of hat/scarf that fits perfectly and has the cutest fabrics.

Idea Number Sixty

Utilize the Internet. There are thousands of websites with information about new drugs, procedures, support groups and clinical trials. I've listed several sites in the back of this book.

Idea Number Sixty-One

Create a drawer or folder with copies of their mammograms, x-rays, doctor writeups and any other information. Everyone needs to be their own patient advocate. It is important to file these in a permanent location. These records should be kept for life. Divide the documents into logical sections to simplify finding a particular document when required.

Idea Number Sixty-Two

Second opinions are a good thing. Working through the different options is overwhelming. It is important that your loved one takes the time, within reason, to think out what is best for them. These are tough choices and what is right for some of us is not necessarily the best choice for others. The best thing you can do is to listen, validate their fears and help with fact gathering. Sometimes it helps to hook up with cancer survivors who have already faced chemotherapy or radiation to discuss side effects and the different choices.

Idea Number Sixty-Three

Some areas have Cancer Boards where your case is reviewed and suggestions are made. These panels have experts in several different fields and can look at the big picture. It seems that each Doctor has tunnel vision, as they should, for their particular area of responsibility. These teams have oncologists, surgeons, radiation oncologist, plastic surgeons and other specialist who can each bring their expertise to the table. Find out if your area has a cancer board and set up an appointment for your loved one.

Idea Number Sixty-Four

Meditation is a great thing to learn and use. Breathing is an amazing thing. Through several of the alternative treatments I learned to use breathing to help deal with pain. There are tapes or classes that you can sign your friend up for or purchase that will teach these methods. Take the class or watch the tapes with them. Breathing also helps stress and who doesn't have that in their lives?

Idea Number Sixty-Five

Clinical trials are in need of cancer patients at different stages of healing. This sometimes helps a person feel like at least something good can come out of having cancer. Help your friend find out about trials in your area. Call the American Cancer Society or check on the Internet.

Idea Number Sixty-Six

Music is a great thing too. Make a tape with their favorite songs they can listen to while driving to appointments, receiving chemotherapy or resting. With CD writers we can now compile tapes or CDs with only their favorite songs. I love Hawaiian music and have a couple of tapes that are just perfect for me.

Idea Number Sixty-Seven

Bring over a baby or a puppy or a kitten if you have one available. New life is very reaffirming, and no one can play with a puppy and not laugh.

Idea Number Sixty-Eight

If the cancer appears to be terminal, help them to create a to do list of things they've always wanted to do and try and help them to complete these things. There are agencies that can help with these wish list. Involve the whole family, give each person a part in making these dreams come true.

Idea Number Sixty-Nine

Plant a special tree, a favorite flower, make a sign or bench with their name on it. Make a party out of it. Picnic lunch, some paint, brushes, and poster paper makes for a great sign. You can also create great posters or banners on the computer.

Idea Number Seventy

Talk openly about what they'd like done after they've passed on. It is comforting to know that things are under control. That there is a plan for the children. It is so difficult to make decisions while dealing with the loss of a loved one. All of us should write down what we would like to have happen to us after our deaths. Anything we can take care of now is going to remove one more burden your loved ones will have to deal with. It is important to have a will and a living will on file. Don't make your family make these decisions. Do it now while you are young and healthy. If there are certain things you really would like to give to certain people, put it in your will. Although my mother had written on the bottom of many things which child should receive her cherished items and told us over the years, this was not carried out upon her death. These items were sold and can never be retrieved.

Idea Number Seventy-One

Utilize Hospice, they are a God send. The great thing about Hospice is they help the entire family. Face it Cancer effects everyone in the home. They can help in obtaining hospital beds, wheelchairs or other special equipment. They also handle nursing care, meals, and emotional support.

Many Cancer patients and their families do not want to face death so they refuse to call in Hospice. Be respectful, but try and prepare them for the reality that they may not survive the Cancer.

This sometimes forces people to prepare for death. Make amends, settle long standing petty grievances and allow the family to say good-bye properly to their loved one.

Idea Number Seventy-Two

Make up a special photo album with all their favorite things, places, and people. With the invention of digital cameras we can all create works of art on our computers.

Idea Number Seventy-Three

Don't be afraid to tell them about the good things going on in your life. Sometimes it's uplifting to know the world is still on track.

Idea Number Seventy-Four

Take pictures of them, and record their voices. Especially people with small children so they'll be able to remember their parent when they were strong and healthy.

Idea Number Seventy-Five

Swimming was one of the few exercises that felt good throughout most of my treatments. Get a pass for them, or go swimming with them somewhere near by. Water aerobics are offered at YMCA pools and most health clubs. You don't necessarily need to be a member to get a special card to just attend these classes.

Idea Number Seventy-Six

Let them know how proud you are and how amazing they are for getting through a tough time. I couldn't hear this enough. Sometimes I would get so down on myself because I ran out of spunk before I got half way through a project I could do before with my eyes closed. Remind them that most of the cures for cancer are a form of poison. You can't expect to be your old self while undergoing these treatments. Enjoy the days they feel great, simplify life so the days they don't feel on top of the world can be spent watching movies, reading, or resting.

Idea Number Seventy-Seven

Any kind of contact is better than no contact at all. Even if you wake them up, or they ask if they can call you back, it is a lonely disease and it is so nice to hear from a friend.

Idea Number Seventy-Eight

Make a donation to one of the many cancer support and or research agencies in their name. Let them know that you think it is an important cause.

Idea Number Seventy-Nine

Figure out what they need close to them and create a little carry all so they can move from the bed to the couch, or sit outside and still have whatever they might require. Phone, water bottle, book, pain medications or anything else they are constantly getting up to retrieve.

Idea Number Eighty

Buy a new set of sheets or bedspread. Or add something new to a room to keep the boredom out. Can't get enough color. Change is good, especially if your bed ridden. Do something to make the room look different each week.

Idea Number Eighty-One

During chemotherapy and radiation your body goes through a cycle. This cycle is different for all of us. I found during radiation Saturdays were my worst day and Sundays were my best. Once I realized this I made sure to keep Saturdays open and tried to plan family events and such on Sundays.

Idea Number Eighty-Two

While they're in having chemotherapy, or surgery decorate the car so when they come out they see something to laugh at. No vandalism, just fun stuff that does not require any cleanup.

Idea Number Eighty-Three

Make a big deal out of their first day back to work. Decorate their desk, plan a luncheon, send them flowers.

Congratulate them and remind them to take it easy.

Idea Number Eighty-Four

Some people, unlike myself want very few people to know they have cancer. Make sure you respect their wishes and if you are one of the few to be let in, make sure you try extra hard to be there for them.

Idea Number Eighty-Five

Take them to a movie or play. It is great to escape for a couple of hours. A good comedy or drama or even an old classic that can distract them from their own troubles and daily tramas.

Idea Number Eighty-Six

Take them for a drive, just to get out of the house for a short time can be very helpful. My husband would let me ride along sometimes when he took our dog for a run. He would park so I had a great view of our dog, Zar running after her ball.

Idea Number Eighty-Seven

If they need to look into special bras or are looking into reconstructive surgeries; contact local cancer agencies in your area for suggestions on what to ask, suggested doctors or stores. There are many catalogs or websites where these items can be purchased without having to leave your home.

Idea Number Eighty-Eight

Once a week e-mail or call their circle of friends or family to give them updates and let them know what they can do to help. Most families are spread out across the country these days.

Idea Number Eighty-Nine

Blow up favorite pictures and keep them close by. I had pictures of my mom, my little sister and my husband and dog that would cheer me up when I was home alone.

Idea Number Ninety

Read out loud to them from the Bible or a favorite book. I love to hear my little sister read to me. I have a devotional that my husband and I read from each night. I really cherish this special time for the two of us each evening.

Idea Number Ninety-One

I really enjoyed having pedicures, or soaking my feet in special oils. Foot massages are soothing also. Get a cute wicker basket and fill it with assorted oils, lotions and exotic doo dads and what nots. You can also offer to give them a massage or pedicure. If your don't have the time or energy to do it yourself, many nail salons sell gift certificates for such treatments.

Idea Number Ninety-two

There is nothing like a bath. Add some special bubbles, favorite music, some candle light. A gift basket works great for this also. I love getting special fragrant bath oils, candles, or even body paints! If the Cancer patient is your significant other, offer to bath them or join them. Make them feel like they are the most beautiful person on the face of the earth.

Idea Number Ninety-Three

There are many many different medications and recommendations for helping with hot flashes. Stop by a health food stores and pick up alternative hot flash remedies. Make sure you verify with their doctor or pharmacy that the drug will not interact adversely with Tamoxifen. Keep trying until they find the right combo. If they are taking Tamoxifen, it eliminates estrogen in the body. Many hot flash medications can not be taken while using Tamoxifen. Their oncologist can also prescribe different medications that will reduce hot flashes.

Idea Number Ninety-Four

Buy a portable fan they can wear around their neck. My husband got me two and I use the heck out of them. Hot flashes always come as the most inopportune times.

Idea Number Ninety-Five

Give them re-sealable moistened wipes for unexpected hot flashes. Part of my job is to teach on the road and I'm sometimes sent to very warm climates. I keep a few in a ziplock and run into the restroom on my breaks and refresh myself.

Idea Number Ninety-Six

Plant seeds at the beginning of the journey and see how they mature just like them. It is amazing how many things I've gained from going through cancer. You would never believe this in the beginning but many good things have come from my experience. I don't take life for granted, I have improved my life style, I remember to tell my loved ones how important they are, and I've gotten my priorities straight.

Idea Number Ninety-Seven

Set up a late afternoon card or board game to play once a week. Just for an hour. This is a great way to get together and catch up.

Idea Number Ninety-Eight

Pray with them or their spouses for guidance and strength. Get on a prayer chain. I even received a piece of fabric from my aunt in Louisiana that her church had prayed over. I brought this with me for my third surgery. It gave me a sense of well being to know I had it pinned to my gown.

Idea Number Ninety-Nine

Help send out thank you notes. There were so many people who did things for me. I was sending out a couple of thank you cards weekly.

Idea Number One Hundred

Arrange for a beauticians to come to their house and do their hair. This is a great treat. Even if it is just a wash and conditioning.

Idea Number One Hundred and One

Just let them know you love them and your there for them. My husband tells me and more importantly shows me how much he loves me every day of my life. With his love I can face most anything life throws at me.

Biblography

American Cancer Society Consumers Guide to Cancer Drugs
Gail M. Wilkes, Terri B. Ades, and, Irwin Krafoff M.D
Jones and Bartlet, October 1999

Beating Cancer with Nutrition: Combining the Best of Science and
    Nature for Healing in the 21st Century with Cdrom
Patrick Quillin,With Noreen Quillin
Nutrition Times Press, Incorporated, January 2001

Bosom Buddies
Rosie O'Donnell and Deborah Axelrod M.D., F.A.C.S.
Warner Books Publishing, 1999

Chicken Soup for the Unsinkable Soul, 101 Inspirational Stories of
    Overcoming Life's Challenges
Jack Canfield, Mark Victor Hansen and Heather McNamara
Health Communications Publishing, 1999

Dr. Susan Love's Breast Book
Susan Love, MD, Breast Surgeon
Addison Wesley Publishing, 1991

Everyday Strength; a Cancer Patient's Guide to Spiritual Survival
Randy Becton
Baker Books, June 1999

Every Woman's Guide To Breast Cancer
Vickie L. Seltzer, MD
Penguin Viking, 1989

Finding a Lump in Your Breast
Judy C. Kneece, RN, OCN
EduCare Publishing, January 1996

Helping Your Mate Face Breast Cancer
Judy C. Kneece, RN, OCN
EduCare Publishing, February 2001

Hyperion, January 2001
Helping Your Mate Face Breast Cancer
Judy C. Kneece, RN, OCN
EduCare Publishing, 1999 3rd Edition

How to Live Between Office Visits
Bernie S. Siegel, M.D.
Harper Collins Books, 1993

Ice Bound: A Doctor's Incredible Battle for Survival at the South Pole
Jerri Nielsen
November 1999

Invisible Scars
Mimi Greenberg, Ph.D.
Walker and Company, 1988

Living beyond Breast Cancer: A Survivor's Guide for when Treatment
Ends and the Rest of Your Life Begins

Marisa C. Weiss,Ellen Weiss
Crown Publishing Group, September 1998

Love, Medicine and Miracles
Bernie S. Siegel, M.D.
Harper and Row, 1996

Mosbys Medical, Nursing and Allied Health Dictionary
Kenneth N. Anderson, Lois E. Anderson and Walter D. Glanze
November, 1997

Natures's Pharmacy In consultation with the American Association of
    Naturopathic Physicians
Publications International, Ltd., 2001

It's Not About the Bike: My Journey back to Life
Lance Armstrong and Sally Jenkins
Berkley Publishing Group, September 2001

John Hopkins Family Health Book: The Essential Home Medical
    Reference Help You and Your Family Promote Good health and
    Manage Illness
By staff members of the Johns Hopkins Medical Institutions
Harper Collins Publishers, December 1998

Solving the Mystery of Breast Pain
Judy C. Kneece, RN, OCN
EduCare Publishing, June 1996

Spinning Straw Into Gold: Your Emotional Recovery From Breast
    Cancer

Ronnie Kaye, MFCC
Simon & Schuster, 1991

Surviving The Storm poems
Patrick W. Flanigan, M.D.
Pacific Grove Publishing, 1999

Tamoxifen and Breast Cancer Second Edition
Michael W. DeGregorio and Valerie j. Wiebe
Yale University Press, 1999

The Breast Cancer Companion
Kathy LaTour
William Morrow and Company, 1993

The Essential guide to Prescription Drugs 2001: Everything You need to
    Know for safe Drug Use
James J. Rybacki and James W. Long
Harper Collins publishers, December 2000

The Menopause Self Help Book Revised 4th Edition
Susan M. Lark, M.D.
Celestial Arts, 1998

The Pocket Guide to Prescription Drugs (PDR)
Pocket Books, 1998

The Race Is Run One Step At A Time:
    My Personal Struggle And Every Woman's Guide To
Taking Charge of Breast Cancer

Nancy Brinker
Simon & Schuster, 1990

The Triumphant Patient
Greg Anderson
Thomas Nelson, 1992

The Yale University School of Medicine Patient's Guide to Medical Test
Faculty members at Yale University School of Medicine
Houghton Mifflin Company, July 1997

The Year ahead 2002: Cancer
Susan Miller
Adobe Acrobat eBook / Barnes & Noble Digital, January 2002

Uplift: Secrets from the Sisterhood of Breast Cancer Survivors
Barbara Delinsky
Pocket Books, September 2001

USP DI, Volume 2, Advice for the Patient: Drug Information in Lay
  Language
United States Pharmacopeia Staff
Medical Economics Company, January 2000

Vitamin Bible For The 21st Century
Earl Mindell's
Warner Books, 1999

WIT
Margaret Edson
Dramatists Play Service, Incorporated, June 1999

The Cancer Dictionary
Roberta Altman and Michael J. Sarg, M.D.

Your Breast Cancer Treatment Handbook:
Judy C. Kneece RN, OCN
EduCare Publishing, 1998 3rd Edition

Your Life in Your Hands: Understanding, Preventing and Overcoming
    Breast Cancer
Jane A. Plant
St. Martin's Press, Inc.,December 2000

SOME USEFUL
ON-LINE REFERENCES
TO BREAST CANCER DIRECTORIES

www.healingwell.com/breastcancer
This site is a very comprehensive & well researched resource center!
Well worth a visit!

www.cancerhelp.com
You'll find lots of detailed information available here. It is very geared
to getting accurate information to the public.

http://www.cancerhelp.com/ed/glossary.htm
Very valuable for any cancer patient that wants to understand what the
heck the doctor is talking about! Hundreds of specialized terms associated with breast cancer are defined in terms the average person can
actually grasp! This site is very worth the visit!

www.wellnessbooks.com/breastcancer
This one offers a wide range of books on the subject of breast cancer.
It's a great way to shop for books without having to leave home.

www.acor.org
This site offers information galore, and even has on-line support
groups! It's a huge non-profit site. Don't miss it!

www.patientcenters.com/breastcancer
This site is especially geared to the patient who has metastatic breast cancer. It has up to date information and explanations of difficult to understand aspects of the disease.

www.blackwomenshealth.com
Committed to getting the best possible information out there to black women and their family and friends, in the most comfortable and familiar way possible. A top notch resource center for the African-American women, but great information is also relevant to non-blacks, so it is a worthy visit for anyone.

www.alphacancer.com
This site is sponsored by the National Cancer Institute. Along with lots of good information, there are on-line audio and visual broadcasts on a variety of cancer issues.

www.blochcancer.org
This is a second opinion center. It gets into the latest experimental treatments, as well as the latest protocols.

www.breastdiseases.com
Treatment options, post-op care and possible complications are the focus of this site. A good way to get the nitty gritty. Knowledge is power, a great man once said.

www.nawho.org
This site is geared to screening Asian women. Or women of Asian descent. It is sponsored by the National Asian Women's Health Organization.

www.kidscope.org.
A videotaped discussion between a mother with breast cancer and her child. It maybe useful in trying to explain to a child you know about what the disease is.

www.lymphnet.org
This site is sponsored by the National Lymphedema Network (NLN) This is where you will find , complete , in-depth information about the whole lymph node issue. Very in-depth and accurate.

www.preventcancer.org
On this site you can even access Spanish language programs, discussing early detection, mammograms, exams, lifestyle, and lots more interesting information.

www.patientadvocate.com
If you need legal advice regarding nursing care or insurance type issues, this is the site to visit. It is sponsored by the Patient Advocate Foundation, or P.A.F.

www.xensicom/users/mjinfo
This site is sponsored by the Mary Jo Nugent Foundation, and it is dedicating to getting financial support to disadvantaged cancer victims and family members.

www.sharecancersupport.org
This site give loads of self-help advice to women and their loved ones, affected by cancer. It has most information in both Spanish and in English. You'll find lots of support groups and information sharing here!

www.needymeds.com

This site is sponsored by a pharmaceutical corporation, but it tries to link you up with organizations that can give you possible financial assistance to purchase expensive medications, should you not have sufficient (or any) insurance to cover it.

www.azstarnet.com/~pud/msdbc

This site caters to the needs of mothers whose daughters have been diagnosed with breast cancer. It was started by a mother who went through this with her daughter. It offers an on-line newsletter and so much more.

www.mediconsult.com

This site offers a site with a glossary of terms related strictly to chemotherapy radiation.

www.lookgoodfeelbetter.org

This site is a great place to go to find out ways to make yourself do just what the title says: Look good, and feel better! It's all free and it's all worth checking out.

www.lbbc.org

This site offers help for young survivors. It includes support groups and lots of chat lines, hotlines, and outreach programs. It's sponsored by Living Beyond Breast Cancer.

www.thebreastclinic.com

This site is very comprehensive and answers many frequently asked questions about issues of breast cancer. It's got loads of information and plenty of links to other great sites.

www.cansearch.org

This site deals with the techniques that have been helpful to others in dealing with surviving cancer treatments. It offers tutorial and coaching.

www.surgery.wisc.edu/wolberg

This site has a Whopper Sized name, so stand back; The Breast Cancer Resources Benign Breast Disease and Breast Cancer Tutorial. (Whew!) But it is a great site to check out that was put together by a woman who is a doctor and she has had breast cancer.

www.yana.org

This site is specially geared to the needs of high-dose chemotherapy. Those of you who may have to go through that, would understand the need of a special support group for that level of treatment. The letters in the name stand for You Are Not Alone.

http://www.hslc.org/emb/bctoc.html

This site talks about getting insurance coverage for high-dose chemotherapy. It also goes into the same for autologous bone marrow transplantation (also known as ABMT/BCT)

http://cancer.med.upenn.edu/disease/breast

This is a University of Pennsylvania Medical dept. It offers very comprehensive information on the disease.

http://www.plasticsurgery.org/surgery/brstrec.htm

If you are thinking of having any plastic surgery after the breast surgery, then it's a good idea to come to this site. If you know someone who is considering it, steer them here before they make the final decision. If they need someone to discuss it with, open your heart and your ears and let them ask your opinion.

www.ibcresearch.org

This site was started by victims of inflammatory breast cancer and is catered strictly to their particular needs. You'll find lots of information and updates here.

www.cancercare.org

This site is dedicated to getting free, professional assistance to people and their families with ANY type of cancer. They help to arrange to get care of all kinds. This site is a must see for anyone who needs help in caring for an cancer patient. It offers information and assistance in Spanish as well as in English. You can even participate in on-line tele-conference educational seminars!

www.nabco.org

This site is sponsored by the National Alliance of Breast Cancer Organizations (NABCO)
On this site you can narrow your search, state by state, to find local care and support in your area.

http://www.usnews.com/usnews/nycu/health/hehome.htm

There is a listing here of the "Best Hospitals in America" . Check it out to see if there is a great one that you can get access to.

http://home.earthlink.net/~rkupbens/mcabc

This site is a men's support group that deals with what the effects of the disease have on their lives, and strives to help them to understand and accept what it does to the woman in their life that suffers from the disease. If you know of anyone that could benefit from this site, it's a great place to send them. It was started by the Men's Crusade Against Breast Cancer, at the Georgetown University Hospital in Washington D.C.

www.cancerlinks.org
Just as the address implies, this site offers multitudes of links to other sites related to cancer issues of all kinds and the various aspects from every angle. There is definitely something for everybody here. This site is a sure Must See.

www.pgh.auhs.edu/bfisher
An oncology professor at the University of Pittsburgh, offers this site to keep you or your loved ones up to date on the latest in cancer research and developments. This site is very much worth a visit. There is a wealth of current information to see here.

www.avoncrusade.com
This is an Avon Breast Cancer Awareness Crusade site that is particularly focused on getting care to cancer patients that advocacy. They award organizations that make efforts to encourage early detection education and services, they do a lot of wonderful things, to numerous to mention here, but they offer a great deal of helpful information and support groups as well.

www.aicr.org
This is an American Institute for Cancer Research site that stresses many great ways to prevent cancers especially through dietary means and the elimination of pesticides and such in the daily intake. There is a wonderful quantity of good information here.

Glossary

This is a copy of the wonderful glossary of terms located on the *www.cancerhelp.com* website.

Abscess
A collection of pus from infection.

Acini
The parts of the breast gland where fluid or milk is produced (singular: acinus).

Acute
Occurring suddenly or over a short period of time.

Adenocarcinoma
A form of cancer that involves cells from the lining of the walls of many different organs of the body. Breast cancer is a type of adenocarcinoma.

Adjuvant Treatment
Treatment that is added to increase the effectiveness of a primary treatment. In cancer, adjuvant treatment usually refers to chemotherapy, hormonal therapy or radiation therapy after surgery to increase the likelihood of killing all cancer cells.

Alkylating Agents
Type of chemotherapy drug used in cancer treatment.

Alopecia
Refers to hair loss as a result of chemotherapy or radiation therapy administered to the head. Hair loss from chemotherapy is
temporary. Hair loss from radiation is usually permanent.

Amenorrhea
The absence or discontinuation of menstrual periods.

Analgesic
Medicine given to control pain; for example: aspirin or Tylenol."

Anesthesia
Medication that causes entire or partial loss of feeling or sensation.

Androgen
A male sex hormone. Androgens may be used in patients with breast cancer to treat recurrence of the disease.

Aneuploid
The characteristic of having either fewer or more than the normal number of chromosomes in a cell. This is an abnormal cell.

Anorexia
Severe, uncontrolled loss of appetite.

Antiemetic
A medicine that prevents or relieves nausea and vomiting, used during and sometimes after chemotherapy.

Antimetabolites
Anticancer drugs that interfere with the processes of DNA production, thus preventing cell division.

Areola
The circular field of dark colored skin surrounding the nipple.

Aspiration
Removing fluid or cells from tissue by inserting a needle into an area and drawing the fluid into the syringe.

Asymptomatic
Without obvious signs or symptoms of disease. Cancer may cause symptoms and warning signs; but, especially in its early
stages, cancer may develop and grow without producing any symptoms.

Atypical Cells
Not usual; abnormal. Cancer is the result of atypical cell division.

Autologous
Coming from the same person.

Axilla
The armpit.

Axillary Dissection
Surgical removal of lymph nodes from the armpit. This tissue is then sent to the pathologist to determine if the breast cancer has
spread outside of the breast. The number of nodes dissected varies during surgery. Your physician can tell you how many
nodes were removed.

Axillary Nodes
The lymph nodes in the axilla (underarm) that are cut out and examined during surgery to see if the cancer has spread past thebreast. The number of nodes in this area varies.

Benign Tumor
An abnormal growth that is not cancer and does not spread to other parts of the body.

Bilateral
Pertains to both sides of the body. For example, bilateral breast cancer would be on both sides of the body or in two breasts.

Biological Response Modifier
Treatment used which alters the body's natural response to stimulate bone marrow to make specific blood cells. Referred to as
colony stimulating factors.

Biopsy
The surgical removal of a small piece of tissue or a small tumor for microscopic examination to determine if cancer cells are
present. A biopsy is the most important procedure in diagnosing cancer.

Biotherapy
Treatments used to stimulate the body's immune system.

Blood Count
A test to measure the number of red blood cells (RBCs), white blood cells (WBCs) and platelets in a blood sample.

Bone Marrow
The soft, fatty substance filling the cavities of the bones. Blood cells are manufactured in the bone marrow. Chemotherapy will
affect the bone marrow, resulting in a temporary decrease in the number of cells in the blood.

Bone Marrow Biopsy and Aspiration A procedure in which a needle is inserted into the center of a bone, usually the hip, to

remove a small amount of bone marrow for microscopic examination.

Bone Scan

The injection of a trace amount of radioactive substance into the bloodstream to illuminate the bones under a special camera to

see if the cancer has spread to the bones.

Breast Cancer

If not removed from the body, a potentially fatal tumor because of its ability to leave the breast and go to other vital organs andcontinue to grow. These are uncontrolled breast cells that are abnormal with uncontrolled growth.

Breast Implant

A round or teardrop shaped sac inserted into the body to restore the shape of the breast. May be filled with saline water orsynthetic material.

Breast Self-Exam (BSE)

A procedure to examine the breasts thoroughly once a month to detect any changes or suspicious lumps. Exams should be

practiced at the end of the period or seven days after the start of the period and be performed monthly at the same time.

Calcifications

Small calcium deposits in breast tissue seen on mammography. The smallest object detected on mammography. Deposits are

the result of cell death. Occurs with benign and malignant changes.

Cancer

A general term used to describe more than 100 different uncontrolled growths of abnormal cells in the body. Cancer cells have

the ability to continue to grow, invade and destroy surrounding tissue, leave the original site and travel via lymph or blood
systems to other parts of the body where they can set up new cancerous tumors.

Cancer Cell
A cell that divides and reproduces abnormally with uncontrolled growth. This cell can break away and travel to other parts of
the body and set up another site, referred to as metastasis.

Clavicle
The collarbone.

Carcinoembryonic Antigen (CEA)
Blood test used to follow women with metastatic breast cancer to help determine if the treatment is working. This is not a test
specific for cancer.

Carcinogen
Any substance that initiates or promotes the development of cancer. For example, asbestos is a proven carcinogen.

Carcinoma
A form of cancer that develops in tissues covering or lining organs of the body, such as the skin, the uterus, the lung or the
breast.

Carcinoma In Situ
An early stage of development, when the cancer is still confined to the tissues of origin. It has not spread outside the area. In
situ carcinomas are highly curable.

CAT Scan or CT Scan
An x-ray view of the body in sections.

Cell
The basic structural unit of all life. All living matter is composed of cells.

Cellulitis
Infection occurring in soft tissues. Your surgical arm has an increased risk for cellulitis because of the removal of lymph nodes.
Pain, swelling and warmth occur in the area.

Chemotherapy
Treatment of cancer by use of chemicals. Usually refers to drugs used to treat cancer.

Clinical Trial
Entering into a cancer treatment program that has proven to be effective after experiments. Evidence has proven potential
effectiveness, and preliminary studies in humans suggest usefulness.

Combination Chemotherapy
Treatment consisting of the use of two or more chemicals to achieve maximum kill of tumor cells.

Combined Modality Therapy
Two or more types of treatments used to supplement each other. For instance, surgery, radiation, chemotherapy, hormonal or
immunotherapy may be used alternatively or together for maximum effectiveness.

Complete Blood Count (CBC)
A laboratory test to determine the number of red blood cells, white blood cells, platelets, hemoglobin and other components of
a blood sample.

Computerized Tomography Scans
Commonly called CT or CAT scans. These specialized x-ray studies indicate cancer or metastasis.

CooperOs Ligaments
Flexible bands of tissue that pass from the chest muscle between the lobes of the breasts, providing shape and support the
breasts.

Core Biopsy
Removal (with a large needle) of a piece of a lump. The piece is sent to the lab to see if the lump is benign or malignant.

Cyst
An abnormal saclike structure that contains liquid or semi-solid material; is usually benign. Lumps in the breast are often found
to be harmless cysts.

Cytology
Study of cells under a microscope that have been sloughed off, cut out or scraped off organs to microscopically examine for
signs of cancer.

Cytotoxic
Drugs that can cause the death of cancer cells. Usually refers to drugs used in chemotherapy treatments.

Detection
The discovery of an abnormality in an asymptomatic or symptomatic person.

Diagnosis
The process of identifying a disease by its characteristic signs, symptoms and laboratory findings. With cancer, the earlier the
diagnosis is made, the better the chance for cure.

Differentiated
The similarity between a normal cell and the cancer cell; defines what degree of change has occurred. Cancer cells that are well
differentiated are close to the original cell and are usually less aggressive. Poorly differentiated cells have changed more and are
more aggressive.

Diaphanography (DPG)
A non-invasive procedure (no cutting) which uses ordinary light as an investigative tool to detect breast masses. Also called
transillumination.

Diploid
The characteristic of having two sets of chromosomes in a cell. This is normal for a breast cell.

DNA
One of two nucleic acids (the other is RNA) found in the nucleus of all cells. DNA contains genetic information on cell growth,
division and cell function.

Doubling Time

The time required for a cell to double in number. Breast cancer has been shown to double in size every 23 to 209 days. It

would take one cell, doubling every 100 days, eight to ten years to reach one centimeter, 3/8 inch.

Ductal Carcinoma In Situ

A cancer inside the ducts of breast that has not grown through the wall of the duct into the surrounding tissues. Sometimes

referred to as a precancer. Good prognosis is involved with in situ cancers.

Ductal Papillomas

Small noncancerous finger-like growths in the mammary ducts that may cause a bloody nipple discharge. Commonly found in

women 45 to 50 years of age.

Edema

Excess fluid in the body or a body part that is described as swollen or puffy.

Endocrine Manipulation

Treating breast cancer by changing the hormonal balance of the body to prevent hormone dependent cancer cells from

multiplying.

Estrogen

A female hormone secreted by the ovaries which is essential for menstruation, reproduction and the development of secondary

sex characteristics, such as breasts. Some patients with breast cancer are given drugs to suppress the production of estrogen in

their bodies.

Estrogen Receptor Assay (ERA)
A test that is done on cancerous tissue to see if a breast cancer is hormone-dependent and may be treated with hormonal
therapy. The test will reveal if your cancer is estrogen receptor positive or negative.

Excisional Biopsy
Surgical removal of a lump or suspicious tissue by cutting the skin and removing the tissue.

Familial Cancer
One occurring in families more frequently than would be expected by chance.

Fat Necrosis Tumor
Destruction of fat cells in the breast due to trauma or injury that can cause a hard noncancerous lump.

Fibroadenoma
A noncancerous, solid tumor most commonly found in younger women.

Fibrocystic Breast Changes or Condition
A noncancerous breast condition in which multiple cysts or lumpy areas develop in one or both breasts. It can be accompanied
by discomfort or pain that fluctuates with the menstrual cycle. Large cysts can be treated by aspiration of the fluid they contain.

Fine Needle Aspiration
Procedure to remove cells or fluid from tissues using a needle with an empty syringe. Cells or breast fluid is extracted by pulling
back on plunger and then is analyzed by a physician.

Flow Cytometry

A test done on cancerous tissues that shows the aggressiveness of the tumor. It shows how many cells are in the dividing stage
at one time, commonly referred to as the "S" phase, and the DNA content of the cancer, referred to as the ploidy. This reveals
how rapidly the tumor is growing.

Frozen Section

A technique in which a part of the biopsy tissue is frozen immediately, and a thin slice is then mounted on a microscope slide,
enabling a pathologist to analyze it in just a few minutes for a diagnosis.

Frozen Shoulder

Surgical shoulder which has severely restricted range of motion and is painful.

Galactocele

A clogged milk duct, often associated with childbirth.

Genes

Located in the nucleus of the cell, genes contain hereditary information that is transferred from cell to cell.

Genetic

Refers to the inherited pattern located in genes for certain characteristics.

Hematoma

A collection of blood that can form in a wound after surgery, an aspiration or from an injury.

Hormonal Therapy

Treatment of cancer by alteration of the hormonal balance. Some cancer will only grow in the presence of certain hormones.

Hormone
Secreted by various organs in the body, hormones help regulate growth, metabolism and reproduction. Some hormones are
used as treatment following surgery for breast, ovarian and prostate cancers.

Hormone Receptor Assay
A diagnostic test to determine whether a breast cancer's growth is influenced by hormones or if it can be treated with
hormones.

Hot Flashes
A sensation of heat and flushing that occurs suddenly. May be associated with menopause or some medications.

Hyperplasia
An abnormal excessive growth of cells that is benign. Intramuscular (I.M.)
To receive a medication by needle injection into the muscle of the body.

Immune System
Complex system by which the body protects itself from outside invaders which are harmful to the body.

Immunology
Study of the body's mechanisms of resistance against disease or invasion by foreign substances. The ability of the body to fight
a disease.

Immunotherapy
A treatment that stimulates the body's own defense mechanisms to combat diseases such as cancer.

Immunosuppressed
Condition of having a lowered resistance to disease. May be a temporary result of lowered white blood cells from
chemotherapy administration.

Incisional Biopsy
A surgical incision made through the skin to remove a portion of a suspected lump or tissue.

Inflammation
Reaction of tissue to various conditions which may result in pain, redness or warmth of tissues in the area.

Infiltrating Cancer
Cancer that has grown through the cell wall of the breast area, in which it originated, and into surrounding tissues.

Informed Consent
Process of explanation to the patient of all risks and complications of a procedure or treatment before it is done. Most informed
consents are written and signed by the patient or a legal representative.

Intraductal
Residing within the duct of the breast. Intraductal disease may be benign or malignant.

Invasive Cancer
Cancer that has spread outside its site of origin and is growing into the surrounding tissues.

In Situ
In place, localized and confined to one area. A very early stage of cancer.

Infiltrating Ductal Cell Carcinoma
A cancer that begins in the mammary glands and has spread to areas outside the gland.

Intravenous (I.V.)
Entering the body through a vein.

Inverted Nipple
The turning inward of the nipple. Usually a congenital condition; but, if it occurs where it has not previously existed, it can be a
sign of breast cancer. Lactation
Process of being able to produce milk from the breasts.

Lesion
An area of tissue that is diseased.

Leukocyte
A white blood cell or corpuscle.

Leukopenia
A decrease in the number of white blood cells, resulting in susceptibility to infection.

Linear Accelerator
A machine that produces high energy x-ray beams to destroy cancer cells.

Liver Scan
A way of visualizing the liver by injecting into the bloodstream a trace dose of a radioactive substance which helps visualize the
organ during x-ray.

Lobular
Pertaining to the part of the breast that is furthest from the nipple, the lobes.

Localized Cancer
A cancer still confined to its site of origin.

Lump
Any kind of abnormal mass in the breast or elsewhere in the body.

Lumpectomy
A surgical procedure in which only the cancerous tumor and an area of surrounding tissue is removed. Usually the surgeon will
remove some of the underarm lymph nodes at the same time. This procedure is also referred to as a tylectomy.

Lymphatic Vessels
Vessels that remove cellular waste from the body by filtering through lymph nodes and eventually emptying into the vascular
(blood) system.

Lymph
A clear fluid circulating throughout the body in the lymphatic system that contains white blood cells and antibodies.

Lymph Glands

Also called lymph nodes. These are rounded body tissues in the lymphatic system that vary in size from a pinhead to an olive

and may appear in groups or one at a time. The principal ones are in the neck, underarm and groin. These glands produce

lymphocytes and monocytes (white blood cells which fight foreign substances) and serve as filters to prevent bacteria from

entering the bloodstream. They will filter out cancer cells but will also serve as a site for metastatic disease. The major ones

serving the breast are in the armpit. Some are located above and below the collarbone and some in between the ribs near the

breast- bone. There are three levels of lymph nodes in the underarm area of the breast and another around the breast bone.

Number of nodes varies from person to person. Lymph nodes are usually sampled during surgery to determine if the cancer has

spread outside of the breast area.

Lymphedema

A swelling in the arm caused by excess fluid that collects after the lymph nodes have been removed by surgery or affected by

radiation treatments.

Macrocyst

A cyst that is large enough to be felt with the fingers.

Magnification View

Special enlarged views to magnify an area for greater detail of suspicious finding. Used in mammography.

Magnetic Resonance Imaging (MRI)
A magnet scan; a form of x-ray using magnets instead of radiation. MRI gives a more clearly defined picture of fatty tissue than
x-ray.

Malignant Tumor
A mass of cancer cells. These cells have uncontrolled growth and will invade surrounding tissues and spread to distant sites of
the body, setting up new cancer sites, a process called metastasis.

Mammary Duct Ectasia
A noncancerous breast disease most often found in women during menopause. The ducts in or beneath the nipple become
clogged with cellular and fatty debris. The duct may have gray to greenish discharge, a lump you can feel and can become
inflamed, causing pain.

Mammary Glands
The breast glands that produce and carry milk by way of the mammary ducts to the nipples during pregnancy and breast
feeding.

Mammogram
An x-ray of the breast that can detect tumors before they can be felt. A baseline mammogram is performed on healthy breasts
usually at the age of 35 to establish a basis for later comparison.

Mammotest
Biopsy (stereotactic) performed under mammography while breast is compressed and lesion is viewed by physician. Sample of

lesion is removed using a large core needle and is then sent to lab to determine if it is benign or malignant.

Margins
The area of tissue surrounding a tumor when it is removed by surgery.

Mastalgia
Pain occurring in the breast.

Mastectomy
Surgical removal of the breast and some of the surrounding tissue.

Modified Radical Mastectomy
The most common type of mastectomy. Breast skin, nipple, areola and underarm lymph nodes are removed. The chest muscles
are saved.

Prophylactic Mastectomy
A procedure sometimes recommended for patients at a very high risk for developing cancer in one or both sides.

Subcutaneous Mastectomy
Performed before cancer is detected, removes the breast tissue but leaves the outer skin, areola and nipple intact. (This is not
suitable with a diagnosis of cancer.)

Radical Mastectomy (Halsted Radical)
The surgical removal of the breast, breast skin, nipple, areola, chest muscles and underarm lymph nodes.

Segmental Mastectomy (Partial Mastectomy/Lumpectomy)

A surgical procedure in which only a portion of the breast is removed, including the cancer and the surrounding margin of
healthy breast tissue.

Mastitis
Infection occurring in the breast. Pain, tenderness, swelling, redness and warmth may be observed. Usually related to infection
and will respond to antibiotic treatment.

Menopause
The time in a woman's life when the menstrual cycle ends and the ovaries produce lower levels of hormones; usually occurs
between the age of 45 and 55.

Metastasis
The spread of cancer from one part of the body to another through the lymphatic system or the bloodstream. The cells in the
new cancer location are the same type as those in the original sites.

Microcalcifications
Particles observed on a mammogram that are found in the breast tissue, appearing as small spots on the picture. Usually occur
from calcium deposits caused by death of breast cells which may be benign or malignant. When clustered in one area, may
need to be checked more closely for a malignant change in the breast.

Microcyst
A cyst that is too small to be felt but may be observed on mammography or ultrasound screening.

Micrometastasis
Undetectable spread of cancer outside of the breast that is not seen on routine screening tests. Metastasis is too limited to have
created enough mass to be observed.

Multicentric
More than one origin or place of growth in the breast. These growths may or may not be related to each other.

Myleosuppression
A decrease in the ability of the bone marrow cells to produce blood cells, including red blood cells, white blood cells and
platelets. This condition increases susceptibility to infection and produces fatigue. Needle Biopsy
Removal of a sample of tissue from the breast using a wide-core needle with suction.

Necrosis
Death of a tissue.

Neoplasm
Any abnormal growth. Neoplasms may be benign or malignant, but the term usually is used to describe a cancer.

Nodularity
Increased density of breast tissue, most often due to hormonal changes, which cause the breast to feel lumpy in texture. This
finding is called normal nodularity, and it usually occurs in both breasts.

Nodule
A small, solid mass. Oncogene

Certain stretches of cellular DNA. Genes that, when inappropriately activated, contribute to the malignant transformation of a
cell.

Oncologist
A physician who specializes in cancer treatment.

Oncology
The science dealing with the physical, chemical and biological properties and features of cancer, including causes, the disease
process and therapies.

One-Step Procedure
A procedure in which a surgical biopsy is performed under general anesthesia and if cancer is found, a mastectomy or
lumpectomy is done immediately as part of the same operation.

Oophorectomy
The surgical removal of the ovaries, sometimes performed as a part of hormone therapy.

Osteoporosis
Softening of bones that occurs with age, calcium loss and hormone depletion.Per Orally (P.O.)
To take a medication by mouth.

Palliative Treatment
Therapy that relieves symptoms, such as pain or pressure, but does not alter the development of the disease. Its primary
purpose is to improve the quality of life.

Palpation
A procedure using the hands to examine organs such as the breast. A palpable mass is one you can feel with your hands.

Pathology
The study of disease through the microscopic examination of body tissues and organs. Any tumor suspected of being cancerous
must be diagnosed by pathological examination.

Pathologist
A physician with special training in diagnosing diseases from samples of tissue.

Pectoralis Muscles
Muscular tissues attached to the front of the chest wall and extending to the upper arms. These are under the breast. They are
divided into the pectoralis major and the pectoralis minor muscles.

Permanent Section
A technique in which a thin slice of biopsy tissue is mounted on a slide to be examined under a microscope by a pathologist in
order to establish a diagnosis.

Platelet
A cell formed by the bone marrow and circulating in the blood that is necessary for blood clotting. Platelet transfusions are used

in cancer patients to prevent or control bleeding when the number of platelets have decreased.

Ploidy
The number of chromosome sets in a cell.

Port, Life Port, Port-A-Cath
A device surgically implanted under the skin, usually on the chest, that enters a large blood vessel and is used to deliver
medication, chemotherapy, blood products and also is used to obtain blood samples. A port is usually inserted if a person has
veins in the arm which are difficult to use for treatment or if certain types of chemotherapy drugs are to be given.

Precancerous
Abnormal cellular changes that are potentially capable of becoming cancer. These early lesions are very amenable to treatment
and cure. Also called pre-malignant.

Progesterone
Female hormone produced by the ovaries during a specific time in the menstrual cycle. Causes the uterus to prepare for
pregnancy and the breasts to get ready to produce milk.

Progesterone Receptor Assay (PRA)
A test that is done on cancerous tissue to see if a breast cancer is progesterone hormone dependent and can be treated by
hormonal therapy.

Prognosis
A prediction of the course of the disease—the future prospect for the patient. For example, most breast cancer patients who

receive treatment early have a good prognosis.

Prolactin
Female hormone which stimulates the development of the breasts and later is essential for starting and continuing milk
production.

Prophylactic Mastectomy
Removal of high-risk breast tissue to prevent future development of cancer.

Prosthesis
An artificial form. In the case of breast cancer following mastectomy, a breast form that can be worn inside a bra.

Protocol
A schedule of selected drugs and treatment time intervals known to be effective against a certain cancer. Radiation Therapy
Treatment with high energy x-rays to destroy cancer cells.

Radiation Oncologist
A physician specifically trained in the use of high energy x-rays to treat cancer.

Radiologist
A physician who specializes in diagnoses of diseases by the use of x-rays.

Radiotherapy
Treatment of cancer with high energy radiation. Radiation therapy may be used to reduce the size of a cancer before surgery or
to destroy any remaining cancer cells after surgery. Radiotherapy can be helpful in shrinking recurrent cancer to relieve

symptoms such as pain and pressure.

Recurrence
Reappearance of cancer after a period of remission.

Regional Involvement
The spread of cancer from its original site to nearby surrounding areas. Regional cancers are confined to one location of the
body. Regional involvement in breast cancer could include spread to the lymph nodes or to the chest wall.

Rehabilitation
Programs that help patients adjust and return to full, productive lives. May involve physical therapy, the use of a prosthesis,
counseling and emotional support.

Relapse
The reappearance of cancer after a disease-free period.

Remission
Complete or partial disappearance of the signs and symptoms of disease in response to treatment. The period during which a
disease is under control. A remission, however, is not necessarily a cure.

Retraction
Process of skin pulling in toward breast tissue, often referred to as dimpling.

Risk Factors
Anything that increases an individual's chance of getting a disease such as cancer. The risk factors for breast disease are a first

degree relative with breast cancer, a high fat diet, early menstruation, late menopause, first child after 30 or no children.

Risk Reduction
Techniques used to reduce your chances of getting a certain cancer. For example, reducing your dietary fat may help prevent
breast cancer. S Phase
Test that is performed to determine how many cells within the tumor are in a stage of division.

Sarcoma
A form of cancer that arises in the supportive tissues such as bone, carti- lage, fat or muscle.

Secondary Tumor
A tumor that develops as a result of metastasis or spreads beyond the original cancer.

Secondary Site
A second site in which cancer is found. Example: cancer in the lymph nodes near the breast is a secondary site.

Side Effects
Usually describes situations that occur after treat- ments. For example, hair loss may be a side effect of chemotherapy; fatigue
may be a side effect of radiation therapy.

Staging
An evaluation of the extent of the disease, such as breast cancer. A classifi- cation based on stage at diagnosis which helps

determine the appropriate treatment and prognosis. In breast cancer, it is determined by whether the lymph nodes are involved;

whether the cancer has spread to other parts of the body (through the lymphatic system or bloodstream) and set up distant

metastasis; and the size of the tumor. Five different stages are used in breast cancer with levels in each stage. Stage IV is the

most serious.

Stellate
Appearing on mammography as a star-shape because of the irregular growth of cells into surrounding tissue. May be

associated with a malignancy or some benign conditions.

Stereotactic Needle Biopsy
Biopsy done while breast is compressed under mammography. A series of pictures locate the lesion, and a radiologist enters

information into a computer. The computer calculates information and positions a needle to remove the finding. A needle is

inserted into the lump, and a piece of tissue is removed and sent to the lab for analysis. May be referred to as mammotest or

core biopsy.

Stomatitis
Inflammation of the gastrointestinal tract creating discomfort and a potential for infection. May be caused by chemotherapy

drugs.

Supraclavicular Nodes
The nodes located above the collar bone in the area of the neck.

Tamoxifen
An anti-estrogen drug that may be given to women with estrogen receptive tumors to block estrogen from entering the breast

tissues. May produce menopause-like symptoms, including hot flashes and vaginal dryness. Currently being used with high risk
women in clinical trials to prevent breast cancer and women who have had breast cancer to prevent recurrence.

Thrombocytopenia
A decrease in the number of platelets in the blood, resulting in the potential for increased bleeding and decreased ability for
clotting.

Tissue
A collection of similar cells. There are four basic types of tissues in the body: epithelial, connective, muscle and nerve.

Transillumination
The inspection of an organ by passing a light through the tissues. Transmission of the light varies with different tissue densities.

Tumor
An abnormal tissue, swelling or mass, may be either benign or malignant.

Two-Step Procedure
When surgical biopsy and breast surgery are performed in two separate surgeries. Ultrasound Examination
The use of high frequency sound waves to locate a tumor inside the body. Helps determine if a breast lump is solid tissue or
filled with fluids.

Ultrasound Guided Biopsy
The use of ultrasound to guide a biopsy needle to obtain a sample of tissue for analysis by a pathologist.

0-595-21670-6